Introduction

Here at www.FunctionalLabz.com we believe you can have fun and get in great shape without costly gym memberships and without taking hours out of your day.

We're all about fun, fast, and highly effective functional workouts that help you reach your health and fitness goals without wasting your time.

This book is full of quick, intense, no equipment bodyweight workouts intended to build muscle, burn fat, and improve overall fitness.

Inside you'll find...

- AMRAP's
- Rounds
- Tabata's
- EMOM's
- Timed Intervals
- and more variety to prevent boredom and keep thing interesting.

Have fun, and please feel free to reach out with any questions or feedback.

~Ryan⁇

10 Reasons to Add Bodyweight Exercise to Your Routine

Bodyweight training may sound like an intimidating new exercise fad. However, it's actually fairly straight forward and minimalist. At its most basic, bodyweight exercises are any form of exercise that does not use weights. Also known to some as calisthenics, this style uses the combination of gravity and the participants own bodyweight to provide resistance. This in turn spurs muscle growth and development.

Bodyweight training has its own specialties and offers some unique benefits that many will find more appealing than a traditional weightlifting routine, or a great addition to any training regimen. Read below to learn some of the potential positives and see if this style of training is a good fit for you.

It's Convenient - Obviously, any type of regular workout requires effort and dedication if you want to produce favorable results. A free ride to the ideal body isn't the kind of convenient we're talking about here. However, one of the major benefits to this type of workout is that it can be done nearly anywhere, at any time. Any open space is a potential gym. If you enjoy working out in the fresh air, you can head out to your local park. If you want privacy, you can clear some space in your garage, spare bedroom, or living room to make your own home gym.

It's Functional - No matter what the latest fitness fad tells you, there are many different routes you can take to get in shape. Free weights have their own benefits, for example. However, the advantage of this minimalist approach is an increase in functional fitness. Lifting static weights increases the strength gain and muscle mass in a specific area. Bodyweight exercise has an effect that is more evenly spread with a special focus on the joints and other connective or supportive muscles. This can help increase overall fitness and improve your abilities in simple day-to-day activities. Things like climbing the stairs at work or walking rugged terrain may suddenly start to feel less arduous and stressful. This can lead to a distinctive improvement in the quality of your daily life. Isn't that worth a little sweat?

It's Cheap - That's right, no barbells, dumbbells, or heavy and expensive equipment here. Since bodyweight exercise uses your own bodyweight and the ever-present power of gravity, you don't have to invest large sums of cash on celebrity endorsed equipment or monthly gym membership fees. Bodyweight training includes things like pushups and regular calisthenics. If you have the space and want to start a garage gym you can install a pull-up bar and some plyo boxes. However, some mats and sturdy, low-level furniture might be all you need if you're just starting out and want to workout at home. This makes bodyweight training ideal for beginners and workout enthusiasts alike.

Develop a Better Base - As stated above, while this method might have less to offer in terms of total strength gain, it can promote better physical fitness overall. A functional fitness approach is great for those who simply want to increase their general health, those who are looking to lose weight, and those who want a more balanced physique. Bodyweight training also helps you get in shape by increasing your stamina and endurance over raw strength. This can help you a great deal later on if you ever decide to incorporate more free weights into your workout routine.

Better Technique - Bodyweight workouts often emphasize precision, posture, and technique. This is because without the ability to simply add more weight, users of this method must be inventive. Adding additional leverage or changing angles and positions incrementally increases the force of gravity and thus the level of resistance. Bodyweight teaches you how to get the most out of each rep, stimulating smaller support muscles that other methods might ignore. This helps develop a level of control that translates to a broad range of different activities and promotes a high level of health and fitness.

Great for Beginners - Besides the low cost and convenience factors mentioned above, what makes this method such a good fit for beginners is that it's fairly straight forward. Many of the exercises involved are familiar to most people and easy to pick up. With a little guidance to help maintain good form a new user should have a workable understanding of the basics in a relatively short period of time. And since there are no heavy weights being lifted, the risk of injury due to poor form is lower.

Once a certain level of performance is reached, exercises can get more complex and physically intensive. However, the learning curve for bodyweight training is quite stable and manageable.

This makes it a perfect approach for people who are not veteran workout enthusiasts or gym freaks. In fact, many casual users who are simply interested in weight loss or increasing overall health and fitness find the intensity of gyms and fitness clubs off putting. This training helps users set their own goals and determine their own schedules, all with minimum out of pocket expense and disruption to their daily lives.

More Flexible - Because these routines don't require set-up or equipment they can be done nearly anywhere. Some common movements include pushups, lunges, squats, step ups, and sit ups. What's great about these exercises is that they can be done in nearly any environment. All you need to do stair climbs is a flight of stairs, so they are perfect if you want to workout at home. Otherwise you can throw down a matt and do some push-ups or sit-ups. Alternatively, exercising outdoors can be exhilarating and may even improve your mood, getting your body all the sunlight and fresh air it needs to keep the mind alert and engaged. You can even do certain exercises at the office, provided you have the time and privacy available in your workspace. Getting up to do some light physical activity is a great way to reduce stress and break up the monotony of a working day.

Stronger Core - The complex movements associated with bodyweight training have a particularly positive effect on the bodies core muscles. Your "core" refers to your obliques, lower back, glutes, and pelvic muscles and play a role in supporting and protecting your spine. The core supports muscles throughout the body, both upper and lower. Along with a trimmer physique, a strong core promotes flexibility, range of motion, and breathing. All these elements combine to make workouts safer and more rewarding and to increase the potential for positive gains by enhancing endurance and adaptability.

Weight Loss - Bodyweight workouts are a great choice for those who want to shed some weight. They usually involve complex movements that require multiple muscle groups to work together, resulting in full-body workouts that lead to reaching your weight loss goals even faster. Losing weight, developing a stronger core, and improving your overall fitness make both regular daily activities and workout sessions easier over time, and allow you push harder. This helps you trim down even more by changing your daily routine, a largely overlooked contributor to unwanted weight gain.

Back to Basics - If the modern gym culture or fitness lifestyle seems commercial and unappealing to you, this may be your ideal route to get your best body. Bodyweight exercises are based on long standing physical fitness traditions that existed long before the fancy fitness equipment we see today. Calisthenics were an integral part of the Greek and Spartan military regimen. They were designed to develop both athleticism, precision, and control in soldiers rather than simply raw strength alone. The result was an army of soldiers who could throw javelins with deadly accuracy, march long distances over inhospitable terrain, and fight in tight formations using a variety of tools.

Hopefully by now you have a better idea of what bodyweight training has to offer. Of course, there is no perfect method and each style has its own benefits based on individual goals and limitations. However, if the combination of low cost, space, and time requirements combined with increased results and a more functional and capable body are appealing to you, then bodyweight exercise might be a good fit for you. Visit www.FunctionalLabz.com for more in-depth resources, workouts, routines, and useful information.

<u>How To:</u>

Repeat for __ Minutes Workouts: These workouts are designed to be repeated for the designated amount of time. To increase intensity, track and record how many rounds you can complete in the given time. Try to beat your score the next time you complete the workout.

Complete __ Rounds Workouts: These workouts are designed to be repeated for the given number of rounds. To increase intensity, record how long it takes you to complete the workout. Try to beat your time the next time you complete the workout.

Ladder Workouts: These workouts are designed to be completed in a ladder, meaning you add one more exercise every round. For example, your first round will be the first exercise. Your second round will be the second and first exercises. Your third round will be the third, second, and first exercises, and so on. Your final round will consist of all exercises. To increase intensity, record how long it takes you to complete the workout. Try to beat your time the next time you complete the workout.

Tabata Workouts: Tabata workouts consist of 20 seconds of the given exercise followed by 10 seconds of rest. Complete the given rounds of each exercise before moving on to the next one. For example, complete 8 rounds of tabata squats (20 seconds on / 10 seconds off) before moving on to tabata pushups.

Every Minute on the Minute Workouts (EMOM): These workouts are designed to be repeated every minute, on the minute, for the given number of minutes. After completing the reps, you have the remainder of the minute to rest.

Even/Odd Minute EMOM: These workouts are designed to be repeated every minute, on the minute, for the given number of minutes. In this case, however, all reps of the first exercise are to be completed in the first minute and all reps of the second exercise are to be completed the next minute. After completing the reps, you have the remainder of each minute to rest.

Deck of Cards: For these workouts you will need a deck of cards. Each suit will have an exercise assigned to it. The number on the card represents the number of reps to be performed for the corresponding exercise. Face cards equal 10 reps. A's equal 11 reps.

How to Increase Intensity:

1. Use a timer. Always try to get as much work done as possible in the given time.
2. Log each workout. Log your total rounds, time, reps, etc. Try to beat that total next time you attempt the workout.

AMRAPs

<u>Repeat for 20 Minutes</u>
5 Burpees
10 Pushups
15 Squats
20 Jumping Jacks

<u>Repeat for 20 Minutes</u>
2 Minute Run
20 Walking Lunges
20 Supermans

<u>Repeat for 20 Minutes</u>
10 T-Pushups
20 Alternating Step Ups
30 Bicycle Crunches

<u>Repeat for 20 Minutes</u>
20 Alternating Lunges
10 Up Down Planks
20 Squats
10 Pike Pushups

<u>Repeat for 20 Minutes</u>
20 Alternating Step Ups
30 Mountain Climbers
40 Jumping Jacks

Repeat for 20 Minutes
10 Pushups
10 Sit Ups
10 Wide Pushups
10 Straight Leg Sit Ups
10 Close Pushups
10 Butterfly Sit Ups

Repeat for 20 Minutes
2 Minute Run
20 Sit Ups
20 Supermans

Repeat for 20 Minutes
1 Minute Run
10 Burpees
100 Flutter Kicks

Repeat for 20 Minutes
10 Burpees
20 Step Back Lunges
30 Russian Twists

Repeat for 20 Minutes
10 Single Leg Deadlifts
20 Hip Bridges
30 Mountain Climbers

Repeat for 15 Minutes
15 Burpees
30 Side to Side Reaches
45 Jumping Jacks

Repeat for 15 Minutes
10 V Ups
10 Jump Squats
10 Jump Lunges

Repeat for 15 Minutes
15 Up Down Planks
15 Jump Squats
15 Sit Ups

Repeat for 10 Minutes
10 Burpees
20 Jump Squats

Repeat for 10 Minutes
15 Squats
30 Mountain Climbers

ROUNDS FOR TIME

<u>Complete 5 Rounds of…</u>
2 Minute Run
1 Minute Plank

<u>Complete 3 Rounds of…</u>
15 Wide Pushups
15 Sit Ups
15 Pushups
15 Straight Leg Sit Ups
15 Close Pushups
15 Butterfly Sit Ups

<u>Complete 5 Rounds of…</u>
10 T-Pushups
20 Supermans
10 Pike Pushups
20 Reverse Snow Angles

<u>Complete 5 Rounds of…</u>
20 Alternating Step Ups
30 Mountain Climbers
40 Jumping Jacks

<u>Complete 4 Rounds of…</u>
2 Minute Run
20 Burpees
20 Squats
20 Sit Ups

Complete 4 Rounds of…
25 Jump Squats
25 Dirty Dogs per leg
25 Jump Lunges
25 Donkey Kicks per leg
25 Bicycle Crunches

Complete 7 Rounds of…
1 Minute Run
15 Side Plank Dips Each Side

Complete 3 Rounds of…
15 Squats
20 Lunges
15 Jump Squats
20 Jump Lunges

Complete 4 Rounds of…
15 Jump Squats
15 Close Pushups
15 Jump Squats
15 Wide Pushups

Complete 8 Rounds of…
25 Squats
50 Jumping Jacks

Complete 5 Rounds of…
30 Squats
30 Mountain Climbers

Complete 10 Rounds of…
100 Meter Sprint
10 Push Ups

Complete 5 Rounds of…
30 Squats
20 Push Ups
10 V Ups

Complete 3 Rounds of…
20 Push Ups
20 20 Squats
20 Up/Down Planks
20 20 Jump Squats

Complete 10 Rounds of…
50 Meter Sprint
10 Burpees

Complete 5 Rounds of…
10 Single Leg Burpees
20 Up/Down Planks
30 Reverse Snow Angles

Complete 3 Rounds of…
20 Wide Push Ups
20 Walking Lunges
20 Diamond Push Ups
20 Jump Lunges

Complete 10 Rounds of…
100 Jumping Jacks
10 Squats
10 Push Ups

Complete 8 Rounds of…
100 Meter Sprint
Bear Crawl back to start

Complete 10 Rounds of…
100 High Knees
10 Diamond Push Ups
10 Straight Leg Sit Ups

Complete 4 Rounds of…
15 Push Ups
30 Dirty Dogs per leg
15 Diamond Push Ups
30 Donkey Kicks per leg
30 Flutter Kicks

Complete 10 Rounds of…
50 Meter Sprint
Reverse Bear Crawl back

Complete 2 Rounds
10 Pike Pushups
20 Burpees
30 Squats
40 Alternating Lunges
50 Sit Ups
40 Alternating Lunges
30 Squats
20 Burpees
10 Pike Pushups

Complete 2 Rounds

10 Pull Ups
20 Supermans
30 V Ups
40 Squat Jacks
50 Walking Lunges
40 Squat Jacks
30 V Ups
20 Supermans
10 Pull Ups

Complete 1 Round

5 Minute Run
10 Burpees
20 T-Pushups
30 Sit Ups
40 Walking Lunges
50 Squats
40 Walking Lunges
30 Sit Ups
20 T-Pushups
10 Burpees
5 Minute Run

Complete 2 Rounds

10 Burpees
20 Up/Down Planks
30 Mountain Climbers
40 Squats
50 Reverse Lunges
40 Squats
30 Mountain Climbers
20 Up/Down Planks
10 Burpees

Complete 1 Round

5 Sprints (50 Meters)
10 Burpees
20 Jump Squats
30 Jump Lunges
40 Toe Touches
50 Straight Leg Sit Ups
40 Toe Touches
30 Jump Lunges
20 Jump Squats
10 Burpees
5 Sprints (50 Meters)

Complete 2 Rounds (Core)

10 V Ups
20 Side Plank Dips
30 Side to Side Reaches
40 Flutter Kicks
50 Mountain Climbers
40 Flutter Kicks
30 Side to Side Reaches
20 Side Plank Dips
10 V Ups

Complete 1 Round

5 Minute Run
10 Pull Ups
20 Up/Down Planks
30 Mountain Climbers
40 Flutter Kicks
50 Straight Leg Sit Ups
40 Flutter Kicks
30 Mountain Climbers
20 Up/Down Planks
10 Pull Ups
5 Minute Run

Complete 2 Rounds

10 Jump Squats
20 Jump Lunges
30 Squats
40 Reverse Lunges
50 Hip Bridges
40 Reverse Lunges
30 Squats
20 Jump Lunges
10 Jump Squats

Complete 1 Rounds

5 Minute Run
10 Burpees
20 Up/Down Planks
30 Diamond Push Ups
40 Reverse Snow Angles
50 Push Ups
40 Reverse Snow Angles
30 Diamond Push Ups
20 Up/Down Planks
10 Burpees
5 Minute Run

Complete 1 Round

5 Minute Run
50 Squats
50 Push Ups
50 Walking Lunges
50 Straight Leg Sit Ups
5 Minute Run

Complete 1 Round

3 Minute Run
30 Squats
30 Lunges
2 Minute Run
20 Squats
20 Lunges
1 Minute Run
10 Squats
10 Lunes
2 Minute Run
20 Squats
20 Lunges
3 Minute Run
30 Squats
30 Lunges

Complete 1 Round

3 Minute Run
30 Pushups
30 Supermans
2 Minute Run
20 Pushups
20 Supermans
1 Minute Run
10 Pushups
10 Supermans
2 Minute Run
20 Pushups
20 Supermans
3 Minute Run
30 Pushups
30 Supermans

<u>**Complete 1 Round**</u>
3 Minute Run
30 Sit Ups
30 Toe Touch Crunches
2 Minute Run
20 Sit Ups
20 Toe Touch Crunches
1 Minute Run
10 Sit Ups
10 Toe Touch Crunches
2 Minute Run
20 Sit Ups
20 Toe Touch Crunches
3 Minute Run
30 Sit Ups
30 Toe Touch Crunches

<u>**Complete 1 Round**</u>
100 High Knees
20 Burpees
100 High Knees
40 Push Ups
100 High Knees
60 Squats
100 High Knees
80 Walking Lunges
100 High Knees
60 Squats
100 High Knees
40 Push Ups
100 High Knees
20 Burpees

Complete 1 Round

100 Jumping Jacks
25 Burpees
100 Jumping Jacks
50 Sit Ups
100 Jumping Jacks
75 Walking Lunges
100 Jumping Jacks
100 Squats
100 Jumping Jacks
75 Walking Lunges
100 Jumping Jacks
50 Sit Ups
100 Jumping Jacks
25 Burpees

Complete 50, 40, 30, 20, 10 Reps of…

Jumping Jacks
Sit Ups

Complete 50, 40, 30, 20, 10 Reps of…

Jump Squats
Pushups
Sit Ups

Complete 50, 40, 30, 20, 10 Reps of…

Walking Lunges
Lazy Burpees
Toe Touch Crunches

EMOMs

<u>12 Minute EMOM</u>
5 Burpees
20 Mountain Climbers

<u>12 Minute EMOM</u>
10 Push Ups
20 Squat Jacks

<u>12 Minute EMOM</u>
5 Pull Ups
10 Straight Leg Sit Ups

<u>15 Minute EMOM</u>
5 Burpees
20 Squat Jacks

<u>15 Minute EMOM</u>
10 Up/Down Planks
10 Sit Ups

<u>15 Minute EMOM</u>
4 Pull Ups
8 Burpees

<u>20 Minute EMOM</u>
5 Burpees
10 Alternating Lunges

20 Minute EMOM
5 Burpees
10 Step Back Lunges

20 Minute EMOM
5 Burpees
15 Squats

20 Minute EMOM
5 Burpees
15 Sit Ups

20 Minute EMOM
5 Burpees
12 Jump Lunges

20 Minute EMOM
5 Burpees
12 Jump Squats

20 Minute EMOM (Even/Odd)
10 Burpees (Even minutes)
20 Sit Ups (Odd minutes)

LADDERS

Ladder
5 Burpees
10 Up Down Planks
15 Jump Squats
20 Jump Lunges
25 Sit Ups
30 Mountain Climbers

Ladder
5 Pull Ups
10 Burpees
15 Single Leg Deadlifts
20 Squat Jacks
25 Mountain Climbers
30 Supermans

Ladder
5 Pull Ups
10 V-Ups
15 Up/Down Planks
20 Jump Lunges
25 Squats
30 Burpees

Ladder
5 Burpees
10 Diamond Push Ups
15 Squats
20 Reverse Lunges
25 Supermans
30 Straight Leg Sit Ups

Ladder
10 Diamond Push Ups
20 Straight Leg Sit Ups
30 Reverse Lunges
40 Push Ups

Ladder
10 Burpees
20 Jump Squats
30 Walking Lunges
40 Toe Touches

INTERVAL WORKOUTS

<u>Tabata</u>
Walking Lunges
Push Ups
Squats
Sit Ups

<u>Tabata</u>
Jump Squats
Diamond Push Ups
Jump Lunges
Up/Down Planks

<u>Tabata</u>
Burpees
Mountain Climbers
Supermans
Hollow Rock

<u>Tabata</u>
Push Ups
Reverse Snow Angles
Up/Down Planks
Supermans
Burpees

<u>Tabata</u>
Burpees
Reverse Lunges
Squats
Russian Twists
Flutter Kicks

Tabata
Burpees
Left Foot Hops
Right Foot Hops
Mountain Climbers
Flutter Kicks

3 Rounds
1 Minute Burpees
1 Minute Walking Lunges
1 Minute Jumping Jacks
1 Minute Wall Sit
1 Minute Plank
1 Minute Rest

3 Rounds
1 Minute Skier Hops
1 Minute Plank Jacks
1 Minute Squat Jacks
1 Minute Up/Down Planks
1 Minute Flutter Kicks
1 Minute Rest

3 Rounds
1 Minute Single Leg Burpees (L)
1 Minute Single Leg Deadlift (L)
1 Minute Single Leg Burpees (R)
1 Minute Single Leg Deadlift (R)
1 Minute V Ups
1 Minute Rest

3 Rounds

1 Minute Forward Bear Crawl
1 Minute Walking Lunges
1 Minute Reverse Bear Crawl
1 Minute Squats
1 Minute Flutter Kicks
1 Minute Rest

3 Rounds

1 Minute Burpees
1 Minute Squats
1 Minute Reverse Lunges
1 Minute Push Ups
1 Minute Sit Ups
1 Minute Rest

3 Rounds

1 Minute T-Push Ups
1 Minute Alternating Lunges
1 Minute Lazy Burpees
1 Minute Reverse Snow Angles
1 Minute Plank
1 Minute Rest

3 Rounds (Cardio)

1 Minute Jumping Jacks
1 Minute High Knees
1 Minute Plank Jacks
1 Minute Skier Hops
1 Minute Mountain Climbers
1 Minute Rest

5 Rounds

30sec Dirty Dogs (left)
30sec Dirty Dogs (right)
30sec Donkey Kicks (left)
30sec Donkey Kicks (right)
30sec Up/Down Planks
30sec Burpees
30sec Rest

5 Rounds (Cardio)

30sec Burpees
30sec Plank Jacks
30sec Jumping Jacks
30sec High Knees
30sec Mountain Climbers
30sec Rest

4 Rounds (Upper Body)

30sec Push Ups
30sec Reverse Snow Angles
30sec Up/Down Planks
30sec Supermans
30sec Rest

4 Rounds (Lower Body)

30sec Squats
30sec Lunges
30sec Jump Squats
30sec Jump Lunges
30sec Skier Hops
30sec Rest

CARDS

Deck of Cards
Clubs: Sit Ups
Spades: Push Ups
Diamonds: Squats
Hearts: Lunges
Joker: 100 Mountain Climbers

Deck of Cards
Clubs: Burpees
Spades: Sit Ups
Diamonds: Hip Bridges
Hearts: Reverse Snow Angles
Joker: 200 Jumping Jacks

Deck of Cards
Clubs: V Ups
Spades: Up/Down Planks
Diamonds: Jump Squats
Hearts: Supermans
Joker: 150 Flutter Kicks

Deck of Cards
Clubs: T-Push Ups
Spades: Jump Squats
Diamonds: Burpees
Hearts: Jump Lunges
Joker: 3 Minute Run

Deck of Cards-Lower Body
Clubs: Single Leg Deadlifts
Spades: Calf Raises (x2)
Diamonds: Jump Squats
Hearts: Reverse Lunges
Joker: 100 Toe Hops

Deck of Cards-Lower Body
Clubs: Side Lunges
Spades: Hip Bridges (x2)
Diamonds: Jump Lunges
Hearts: Squats (x2)
Joker: 150 Skier Hops

Deck of Cards-Upper Body
Clubs: Reverse Snow Angles
Spades: Pike Push Ups
Diamonds: Up/Down Planks
Hearts: Push Ups
Joker: 3 Minute Run

Deck of Cards-Upper Body
Clubs: Diamond Push Ups
Spades: Wide Push Ups
Diamonds: Burpees
Hearts: Reverse Snow Angles
Joker: 150 Jumping Jacks

Deck of Cards-Core
Clubs: Left Side V-Ups
Spades: Right Side V-ups
Diamonds: Supermans
Hearts: Straight Leg Sit Ups
Joker: 100 Flutter Kicks

<u>Deck of Cards-Core</u>
Clubs: Right Side Planks
Spades: Left Side Planks
Diamonds: V-Ups
Hearts: Supermans
Joker: 150 Flutter Kicks

THANK YOU

Thank you for purchasing this book. I hope you got what you were looking for out of it. For more workouts, articles, and ideas please visit www.FunctionalLabz.com

Functional Labz